I0768295

Nutritious cuisine for weight loss: "A Guide to Healthy Eating and Sustainable

Dolores E. Flint

Nutritious cuisine for weight loss: "A Guide to Healthy Eating and Sustainable

Disclaimer

Copyright © by Dolores E. Flint 2024. All rights reserved.

Before this document is duplicated or reproduced in any manner, the publisher's consent must be gained. Therefore, the contents within can neither be stored electronically, transferred, nor kept in a database. Neither in Part nor full can the document be copied, scanned, faxed, or retained without approval from the publisher or creator.

Table of Contents

Disclaimer

INTRODUCTION:

Chapter 1: Understanding Nutrition and Weight Loss

Chapter 2: Create a Balanced Plate

Chapter 3: Breakfasts to Start Your Day.

Chapter 4: Delicious Lunches for Busy Days

Chapter 5: Healthy Dinners to Finish Your Day Right

Chapter 6: Snacks to Stay Fueled

Chapter 7: Sweet Treats Without Guilt

Chapter 8: Tips for Dining Out and Social Situations

Conclusion

INTRODUCTION:

Welcome to "Nutritious Cuisine for Weight Loss"! In this book, we'll look at the important link between nutrition and weight reduction, giving you practical insights, delicious recipes, and concrete strategies to help you reach your health and fitness objectives. Whether you're just starting your road to healthy living or seeking new methods to improve your current eating habits, this book will help you every step of the way. Prepare to experience the joy of nourishing your body while losing unwanted pounds, and embark on a revolutionary journey to better health and vitality.

Chapter 1: Understanding Nutrition and Weight Loss

In this foundational chapter, we will look at the essential principles of nutrition and weight loss. Learn about the fundamentals of nutrition, the science behind effective weight loss programs, and how to set realistic goals that are appropriate for your requirements and lifestyle. Understanding the important components of a balanced diet, as well as the elements that lead to successful weight reduction, will enable you to make informed decisions and establish long-term health and wellness habits.

The Basics of Nutrition

In this section, we break down the fundamentals of nutrition, giving you a thorough understanding of the macronutrients and micronutrients that power your body. Learn about how carbohydrates, proteins, and lipids help to maintain energy levels and promote general health. Discover how vitamins and minerals help your body's systems function properly. Armed with this knowledge, you'll be able to make smart food choices, ensuring that your body gets the nutrients it needs to thrive.

The Science Of Weight Loss

Explore the science of weight loss and discover the mechanisms that underlie changes in body composition. Investigate topics like energy balance, metabolism, and the role of hormones in hunger and fat storage. Understand how genetics, environment, and lifestyle behaviors affect weight management. Understanding the physiological processes that drive weight reduction will help you build successful strategies for obtaining and maintaining a healthy body weight.

Setting Realistic Goals

In this section, we will discuss the necessity of creating realistic and achievable goals for your weight loss journey. Learn how to evaluate your existing circumstances, identify your goals, and set measurable targets that are consistent with your lifestyle and preferences. Learn the importance of defining both short-term and long-term objectives, and how breaking them down into achievable steps can improve your chances of achievement. Setting realistic goals will help you build a plan of action and stay motivated as you work toward your desired outcomes.

Chapter 2: Create a Balanced Plate

Discover how to prepare well-balanced meals that nourish your body while also helping you lose weight. Learn the value of including a range of nutrient-dense foods in your diet, such as lean proteins, whole grains, fruits, vegetables, and healthy fats. Discover tactics for portion control and mindful eating to help you maintain a healthy caloric intake. By mastering the skill of creating a balanced plate, you'll maximize your nutrition intake and create the groundwork for long-term weight loss success.

Macronutrients: carbohydrates, proteins, and healthy fats

Explore the world of macronutrients and discover how carbohydrates, protein, and healthy fats play important roles in your diet and weight loss quest. Understand each macronutrient's role in energy levels and general wellness. Discover how to establish the perfect macronutrient balance to help you lose weight while also meeting your nutritional demands. With a better grasp of macronutrients, you'll be able to make smart food choices and prepare meals that feed your body for success.

Carbohydrates :

• Carbohydrates are the main source of energy. These foods include grains, fruits, vegetables, and legumes. Carbohydrates are classified into two types: simple (sugars) and complex (starches and fiber).

• Simple carbs digest fast and might produce sudden rises in blood sugar levels. They can be found in meals such as candy, soda, and baked goods.

• Complex carbohydrates take longer to digest, resulting in a more prolonged energy release. These foods include whole grains, legumes, and veggies. For prolonged energy and superior overall health, complex carbs should always be preferred over simple carbohydrates.

Protein:

• Protein is needed for tissue formation and repair, as well as other physiological activities in the body.

• It is composed of amino acids, which are commonly referred to as the building blocks of proteins.

• Protein-rich foods include lean meats, poultry, fish, eggs, dairy products, tofu, legumes, nuts, and seeds.

• Including protein in meals and snacks can boost satiety, control blood sugar levels, and promote muscle maintenance and growth.

• Aim to include protein in every meal and snack throughout the day to improve overall health and weight loss efforts.

Healthy Fats:

• Healthy fats play crucial roles in supporting brain function, hormone production, and the absorption of fat-soluble vitamins (A, D, E, and K).

• Sources of healthy fats include avocados, nuts, seeds, olive oil, fatty fish (such as salmon and mackerel), and coconut oil.

• Monounsaturated and polyunsaturated fats, found in foods like avocados, nuts, seeds, and fatty fish, are considered healthy fats that can help reduce the risk of heart disease and inflammation.

• It's essential to limit the intake of unhealthy fats, such as trans fats and saturated fats, which are found in processed foods, fried foods, and fatty cuts of meat.

• Including a variety of healthy fats in to your diet can help promote satiety, enhance flavor, and support overall health and well-being.

Balancing your carbohydrate, protein, and healthy fat intake is essential for achieving your weight loss objectives while maintaining ideal nutrition and energy levels. To attain a well-rounded and enjoyable diet, incorporate nutrient-dense foods from each macronutrient group into your meals and snacks.

Micronutrients: vitamins and minerals

Micronutrients, which include vitamins and minerals, are required for many physiological functions in the body, including metabolism, immunological function, and cell repair. Let's examine each one more closely.

Vitamins:

• Vitamins are chemical molecules that the body requires in little doses to function normally.

• Vitamins are classified into two types: water-soluble (vitamins B and C) and fat-soluble (vitamins A, D, E, and K).

• Water-soluble vitamins cannot be stored in the body and must be supplied regularly by diet or supplementation. They have important roles in energy metabolism, immunological function, and neuronal function.

• Fat-soluble vitamins are stored in the body's fat cells and liver and absorbed in conjunction with dietary fat. They are critical for vision, bone health, immunological function, and antioxidant defense.

Minerals:

• Minerals are inorganic substances that the body needs for several physiological functions, including bone formation, fluid balance, and muscle function.

• Minerals are classified into two types: macrominerals (needed in larger proportions) and trace minerals.

• The macro minerals are calcium, magnesium, phosphorus, potassium, sodium, and chloride. They have important roles in bone health, muscular function, nerve transmission, and fluid balance.

• Trace minerals consist of iron, zinc, copper, selenium, iodine, manganese, and chromium. Although in smaller levels, they are required for a variety of processes, including energy synthesis, immunological function, and antioxidant action.

To ensure adequate vitamin and mineral intake:

• Consume a wide variety of fruits, vegetables, whole grains, lean meats, and healthy fats.

• Choose colorful fruits and vegetables for higher vitamin and mineral content. * If you have dietary limitations, nutrient shortages, or special health concerns, you might consider taking a multivitamin or specific vitamins and minerals.

• Cooking processes can impact the nutritional value of meals. Consult a healthcare practitioner or certified dietitian for tailored advice on fulfilling your micronutrient requirements.

Prioritizing a vitamin and mineral-rich diet will improve your general health, optimize biological processes, and help you lose weight.

Portion Control and Mindful Eating

Portion control and mindful eating are crucial habits for weight management and overall health. Here's what you should know.

Portion control: Portion control entails limiting the amount of food you eat at meals and snacks to maintain a healthy calorie balance.

• Portion size is crucial to consider, as larger servings can lead to overeating and obesity.

• Use visual clues or measuring equipment to determine the optimal portion proportions for various dietary groups, such as protein, carbs, and fats.

• Pay attention to the serving sizes given on food labels, and be aware of portion distortion, which occurs when huge restaurant servings or oversized containers affect views of proper quantities.

• Practice portion control by serving yourself smaller servings, using smaller dishes and bowls, and refraining from eating directly from the container.

Mindful eating: Mindful eating entails paying close attention to the sensory experiences of eating, such as taste, texture, fragrance, and contentment.

• Take each bite slowly and relish it, chewing thoroughly and fully experiencing the flavors and textures.

• Eat without distractions, such as television, smartphones, or computers, to concentrate on the act of eating and pay attention to your body's hunger and fullness signals.

• Pay attention to your body's hunger and fullness signals, eating when you're hungry and stopping when you're pleasantly full.

• Be aware of emotional eating triggers and use alternate coping techniques, such as writing, mediation or engaging in enjoyable activities, to address emotional needs without needing food.

By implementing portion management and mindful eating techniques into your daily routine, you may improve your relationship with food, avoid overeating, and manage your weight more effectively. These tactics raise awareness of food choices, improve digestion, and increase overall meal satisfaction, resulting in long-term success in obtaining and maintaining a healthy weight.

Chapter 3: Breakfasts to Start Your Day.

Start your mornings right with a delicious and nutritious breakfast that will energize your body and set a positive tone for the day. In this chapter, we'll look at a selection of breakfast options that will satisfy your cravings while also helping you lose weight. From invigorating smoothie bowls filled with fruits and veggies to protein-packed omelets and frittatas, as well as comforting whole grain porridges and cereals, you'll find plenty of inspiration to start your day on a healthy note. Whether you prefer quick and easy meals or leisurely weekend brunches, these breakfast recipes will become your new favorites. Say goodbye to boring breakfasts and hello to a healthful start to your day!

Energizing Smoothie Bowls

Our collection of revitalizing smoothie bowl recipes will help you find the ideal blend of flavor and nutrition. These vivid and delicious bowls are packed with fruits, veggies, and superfoods to give you a boost of energy. From tropical-inspired mixes with mango, pineapple, and coconut to antioxidant-rich compositions with berries and leafy greens, there's a smoothie bowl for every taste. For extra texture and crunch, sprinkle them with a variety of healthful toppings including nuts, seeds, granola, and fresh fruit. These nutrient-dense smoothie bowls will quickly become a favorite part of your morning routine, whether as a filling breakfast or a refreshing snack. Prepare to fuel your body and nourish your taste senses with these delicious and nutritious recipes.

Protein-Rich Omelets and Frittatas

Our protein-packed omelets and frittatas are ideal for providing long-lasting energy throughout the day. These savory dishes are packed with lean proteins, colorful veggies, and fragrant herbs and spices that will satisfy your taste buds and keep you full until your next meal. Whether you favor traditional combos like spinach and feta or more daring ones like smoked salmon and avocado, there's an omelet or frittata recipe to suit every taste. These flexible recipes are perfect for busy mornings or leisurely brunches, as they require little preparation and offer limitless modification options. Our protein-packed omelets and frittatas will put an end to breakfast dullness and welcome you to a tasty and nutritious start to your day.

Whole Grain Porridges and Cereals

Revitalize your breakfast routine with our hearty and nutritious whole-grain porridges and cereals, ideal for getting your day started right. These nutritional dishes are high in fiber, vitamins, and minerals, and they give continuous energy while keeping you full and satisfied throughout the morning. From creamy oatmeal laced with warming spices and topped with fresh fruit to crunchy granola clusters packed with nuts and seeds, there's a whole-grain porridge or cereal recipe for every taste. Whether hot or cold, sweet or savory, these tasty and healthful selections will quickly become a morning favorite. Say goodbye to processed breakfast cereals and welcome the natural richness of whole grains with our selection of nutritious porridges and cereals.

Chapter 4: Delicious Lunches for Busy Days

Take the worry out of lunchtime with our assortment of filling meals for hectic days. Whether you're working from home, on the go, or simply short on time, these lunch ideas are quick, easy, and flavorful. This chapter has something for everyone, from vivid salads brimming with fresh veggies and protein to tasty soups and stews that warm you from the inside out, as well as nutrient-dense sandwiches and wraps ideal for portability. With minimal preparation and maximum flavor, these filling meals will keep you fuelled and focused as you tackle the remainder of your day. Say goodbye to boring lunches and welcome to tasty and nutritious meals that fit perfectly into your busy schedule.

Vibrant Salad Creations

Elevate your lunchtime experience with our colorful salads that are both delicious and nutritious. These salads are anything but boring, with their vibrant colors and robust flavors. There's a salad dish for everyone's taste, from classics like Caesar and Cobb to imaginative combinations using grains, legumes, and seasonal veggies. To make a tasty and well-balanced dinner, combine crisp greens, crunchy veggies, creamy avocado, pungent cheeses, and protein-rich toppings such as grilled chicken or chickpeas. With handmade dressings and garnishes that provide an added layer of taste, these salads are likely to become a lunchtime staple. With our collection, you can say goodbye to boring salads and hello to a world full of bright flavors and textures.

Flavorful soups and stews

Warm up your lunchtime with our variety of tasty soups and stews, which are ideal for filling your stomach and calming your soul on cold days. From hearty vegetable soups bursting with seasonal produce to rich and aromatic stews loaded with soft meats and lentils, there's a recipe for every taste and dietary desire. These recipes are brimming with flavor and nourishment, having been perfectly seasoned with herbs, spices, and aromatic vegetables. Whether served as a light lunch or combined with a side salad or crusty bread for a more substantial dinner, these soups and stews will warm you from the inside out and leave you feeling nourished and full. Say goodbye to dull lunches and hello to the warm embrace of our delectable soups and stews.

Nutrient-Dense Sandwiches and Wraps

Rethink your lunchtime routine with our assortment of nutrient-dense sandwiches and wraps, which are ideal for powering your day with clean ingredients and delicious flavors. From basic combos like turkey and avocado to new twists like grilled vegetables, hummus, and fresh herbs, there's a sandwich or wrap to satisfy your craving. These handheld meals are packed with lean proteins, colorful vegetables, and whole-grain bread or wraps, making them easy, portable, and nutritious. These nutrient-dense sandwiches and wraps will become your new lunchtime favorites, whether you're searching for a quick and easy choice to eat at your desk or a filling meal to take on the move. Say goodbye to uninspiring lunches and hello to our nutrient-dense concoctions, which are both delicious and nourishing.

Chapter 5: Healthy Dinners to Finish Your Day Right

Finish your day with our assortment of healthy dinner recipes that will fuel your body while also satisfying your taste senses. This chapter has something for everyone, from lean protein entrees to vegetable-packed stir-fries and skillets, as well as healthful one-pot meals. These dishes are ideal for hectic weeknights when you want a quick and easy meal that is both flavorful and nutritious. With basic materials and minimal preparation, you can make great dinners that will leave you feeling full and content. Say goodbye to takeout and welcome homemade goodness with our selection of healthy dinners to round out your day.

Lean protein entrees

Indulge in a delicious evening with our lean protein entrées, designed to fuel your body while tantalizing your taste buds. From luscious grilled chicken and tender fish fillets to flavorful tofu and robust legume-based recipes, there's a protein-packed option to suit every taste. These entrées are packed with nutrients and flavor, making them the ideal centerpiece for a well-balanced meal. Accompanied by vivid veggies, nutritious grains, and tasty sauces, these dishes will leave you feeling filled and satiated without weighing you down. Say goodbye to bland dinners and hello to the delicious goodness of our lean protein entrées, which will leave you feeling satisfied at the end of the day.

Veggie-Packed Stir-Fries and Skillets

Enhance your dinner game with our veggie-packed stir-fries and skillets, which are brimming with beautiful colors, robust flavors, and healthful ingredients. From classic stir-fry combos with crisp vegetables and soft meats or tofu to hearty skillet meals laden with healthful grains, legumes, and seasonal produce, there's a recipe for every taste and dietary preference. These one-pan marvels are excellent for hectic weeknights when you need a quick and easy meal that doesn't sacrifice taste or nutrition. With minimal prep and cleaning, you can quickly prepare a great and enjoyable dinner. Say goodbye to dull dinners and hello to the intriguing tastes of our veggie-packed stir-fries and skillets, which are sure to satisfy your taste buds while nourishing your health.

Nourishing One-Pot Meals

Simplify your dinner routine with our selection of delicious one-pot meals, which are designed to reduce cleanup while increasing flavor and nutrition. These dishes range from soothing soups and stews to hearty casseroles and skillet meals, making them ideal for hectic weeknights when you need a filling supper with little effort. Simply combine all of your ingredients in one pot, let them simmer and meld together, and enjoy a delicious and nutritious dinner with little effort. These one-pot miracles, packed with protein, fiber, and a variety of bright vegetables, are sure to satisfy your hunger while also nourishing your health. Say goodbye to several pots and pans, and hello to the simplicity and convenience of our nutritious one-pot dinners.

Chaptor 6: Snacks to Stay Fueled

Discover a choice of delicious and nutritious snacks to help you stay energized all day. Whether you're looking for something sweet, savory, or crunchy, this chapter has you covered with delightful options that won't undermine your healthy eating plans. There's a snack for every taste and nutritional requirement, from crunchy veggie sticks with creamy hummus to handmade energy bars packed with nuts and seeds and fresh fruit mixed with protein-rich almonds. With basic ingredients and easy preparation, these snacks are ideal for feeding your busy days and satisfying cravings without sacrificing nutrition. Say goodbye to mindless snacking and welcome to nutritious snacks that will keep you nourished and focused all day.

Crunchy Veggie Sticks and Hummus

Satisfy your snack desires with this delicious blend of crunchy veggie sticks and creamy hummus. Simply cut colorful veggies like carrots, cucumbers, bell peppers, and celery into sticks for a delightful crunch. Combine them with a liberal dollop of homemade or store-bought hummus for a protein-packed and delicious dip. This snack is not only delicious but also extremely nutritious, thanks to its high vitamin, mineral, and fiber content. Enjoy it as a lunchtime pick-me-up or as a pre-dinner appetizer to stave off hunger while feeding your body with nutritious ingredients.

Homemade Energy Bars and Bites

Elevate your snack game with these homemade energy bars and bites, packed with wholesome ingredients to keep you fueled throughout the day. Made with a blend of nuts, seeds, dried fruits, and natural sweeteners like honey or dates, these bars and bites are a nutritious and delicious alternative to store-bought snacks. Customize them with your favorite ingredients and flavors, whether it's classic combinations like almonds and dark chocolate or more exotic options like coconut and goji berries. Perfect for on-the-go snacking or as a pre-workout boost, these homemade energy bars and bites are sure to satisfy your cravings while providing a sustained source of energy. Say goodbye to processed snacks and hello to the wholesome goodness of these homemade treats.

Fresh Fruit and Nut Combinations

With these delectable fruit and nut combinations, you may enjoy the natural sweetness of fresh fruit while still getting the satisfying crunch from nuts. Whether you prefer conventional combinations like apple slices with almond butter or more creative pairings like pineapple chunks with cashews, the options are limitless. Enjoy the rich aromas and textures of nature's abundance while benefiting from the nutritional value of these healthy snacks. These fruit and nut combinations are high in vitamins, minerals, fiber, and healthy fats, making them ideal for satisfying your sweet taste and staving off hunger in between meals. Grab a handful for a quick and easy snack on the run, or eat them leisurely for a filling and nutritious treat. Say goodbye to empty calories and hello to the healthy benefits of fresh fruit and nuts.

Chapter 7: Sweet Treats Without Guilt

Indulge your sweet taste guilt-free with our selection of tasty and nutritious snacks. From lighter dessert swaps to fruit-based pleasures and guilt-free baked goodies, these dishes provide delicious alternatives to classic sweets without sacrificing flavor. Whether you want chocolatey richness, fruity freshness, or cozy baked goods, there's a guilt-free way to satisfy them. These sweet delights, made with healthy ingredients and natural sweeteners, are ideal for a lunchtime pick-me-up, after-dinner dessert, or anytime snack. Say goodbye to sugar cravings and hello to the guilt-free enjoyment of our delicious delicacies that nourish your health while also satisfying your soul.

Guilt-free Dessert Swaps

Our collection of guilt-free dessert alternatives will satisfy your sweet taste without leaving you feeling guilty. Enjoy delectable delicacies such as chocolate mousse, cheesecake, and brownies, all created with healthy ingredients and natural sweeteners. Whether you're craving something creamy, chocolatey, or fruity, there's a guilt-free way to indulge them without jeopardizing your healthy eating objectives. These dessert alternatives, which range from avocado chocolate mousse to Greek yogurt cheesecake and black bean brownies, are both flavorful and nutritious. Enjoy a delectable dessert without guilt, knowing that you're nourishing your body with each bite. Say goodbye to empty calories and hello to guilt-free indulgence with these dessert substitutions.

Fruit-Based Dessert Ideas

Embrace the natural sweetness of fresh fruits with our collection of fruit-based dessert recipes. From refreshing fruit salads and skewers to innovative fruit parfaits and sorbets, there are limitless ways to fulfill your sweet taste while being healthy. Experiment with different fruit combinations, textures, and presentation styles to create visually appealing and delectable desserts. Whether you're eating a simple bowl of mixed berries drizzled with honey or a tropical fruit parfait stacked with Greek yogurt and granola, these fruit-based desserts are sure to please your taste receptors while leaving you feeling delighted. Say goodbye to processed sweets and hello to the natural goodness of fruit-based desserts that feed your health while satisfying your taste buds.

Lightened-up Baked Goods

Our collection of lightened-up recipes allows you to enjoy the familiar taste of baked goods without feeling guilty. From muffins and cookies to cakes and bread, these delicacies are produced with healthier ingredients and contain less sugar and fat, allowing you to enjoy your favorite baked products without jeopardizing your health goals. Whether you want warm banana bread, a chewy oatmeal cookie, or a fluffy blueberry muffin, there's a lighter option to meet your needs. With easy substitutions such as whole wheat flour, Greek yogurt, and natural sweeteners like honey or maple syrup, you may enjoy the familiar taste of baked goods while also nourishing your body with each bite. Say goodbye to hefty desserts and hello to lighter, healthier variations of your favorite baked goods.

Chapter 8: Tips for Dining Out and Social Situations

Navigate dining out and social gatherings with ease by following our practical advice and tactics for selecting healthier choices while still enjoying yourself. These ideas can help you keep on track with your health and fitness objectives whether you're eating out, going to a party, or getting together with friends for dinner. From smart menu choices and portion control to resisting temptations and being attentive to your eating habits, you'll learn how to maintain balance and moderation in every social setting. With a little planning and mindfulness, you can enjoy wonderful meals and good company without jeopardizing your progress. With this eating out and social situations advice, you can say goodbye to tension and hello to confidence and happiness in any dining experience.

Making Smart Choices at Restaurants

Master the art of dining out while staying on track with your health and wellness objectives with our restaurant smart choices guide. Learn how to navigate menus, interpret nutrition labels, and choose healthier options that fit your dietary preferences. From choosing dishes high in lean meats, whole grains, and colorful veggies to adjusting meals to meet your specific needs, you'll learn how to enjoy restaurant meals without losing taste or nutrition. Whether you're dining at a fast-food chain, a casual bistro, or a fancy restaurant, these ideas will help you make informed decisions and enjoy your meal guilt-free. Say goodbye to being intimidated by restaurant menus and welcome to dining out with confidence and pleasure.

Navigating parties and gatherings

Navigate social gatherings and parties with ease by following our suggestions and tactics for making healthier choices while having fun. From cocktail parties and potlucks to holiday gatherings and festivities, these strategies can help you stick to your health and wellness goals without feeling deprived. Learn how to prepare ahead, bring your nutritious dish, and make wise choices from the available options. Learn how to regulate portion sizes, practice mindful eating, and respectfully decline meals that do not fit your goals. With a little planning and attention, you may enjoy social gatherings while prioritizing your health and well-being.

Say goodbye to food-related tension and anxiety at parties and gatherings, and hello to confidence and enjoyment in all social situations.

Mindful-Eating Strategies

Accept the practice of mindful eating to foster a healthier relationship with food and improve your general well-being. Learn how to listen to your body's hunger and fullness cues, as well as your senses of taste, smell, and texture, so you may fully enjoy and appreciate each meal. Slow down and savor your meals without distractions like television or smartphones, so you can better connect with the food and the experience of eating. Practice thankfulness for the nourishment your food offers, and let go of any guilt or judgment about eating. Adopting mindful eating habits can help you enjoy your meals more, improve digestion, and make more balanced food choices that support your health and wellness goals. Say goodbye to mindless eating and hello to thoughtful consumption of every meal.

Staying Consistent on Your Journey

Consistency is critical for long-term success in your health and fitness quest. Here are some suggestions to help you maintain consistency:

• **Set realistic goals:** Break down larger ambitions into smaller, more manageable tasks. To keep motivated, celebrate each milestone you reach.

• **Create routines:** Incorporate healthy behaviors into your everyday routine, such as meal planning, regular exercise, and getting enough sleep. Consistency improves as these routines become second nature.

• **Find balance:** Be flexible and balanced in your approach to health. Aim for progress rather than perfection, and allow yourself to indulge on occasion without feeling guilty.

• **Maintain accountability:** Whether it's by charting your progress, joining a supportive network, or working with a coach or accountability partner, find ways to hold yourself accountable to your goals.

• **Self-care:** Set aside time for activities that nurture your body, mind, and spirit. Meditation, spending time outside, or engaging in enjoyable hobbies are all options.

• **Learn from setbacks:** Recognize that setbacks are an expected part of any endeavor. Instead of lingering on them, consider what you can learn from the event and utilize it to propel your future advancement.

• **Maintain a good attitude:** Avoid concentrating on setbacks and instead focus on the progress you've achieved. To stay motivated, surround yourself with positive messages and affirmations.

Staying persistent and committed to your goals will allow you to gradually gain momentum and make long-term improvements that benefit your health and well-being. Remember, every small step forward matters, and you can build the life you want. Keep moving, and you will arrive at your target!

Celebrate Your Successes

It's critical to recognize and appreciate your accomplishments along your health and fitness journey. Celebrating accomplishments, large or small, can enhance motivation and promote healthy behaviors. Here are some methods to celebrate your success:

• **Reflect on your accomplishments:** Take a moment to consider how far you've gone since beginning your adventure. Recognize your progress, whether it's attaining a weight loss goal, increasing your exercise level, or adopting healthy eating habits.

• **Reward yourself:** Give yourself something special as a reward for accomplishing your goals. This might include new exercise gear, a massage, a day trip to your favorite destination, or anything else that makes you happy and relaxed.

• **Celebrate your success:** Share your accomplishments with friends, family, and members of your support network. Celebrating your accomplishments with others can boost your confidence and deepen your commitment to your goals.

• **Take photos or keep a journal:** Use photos or journal entries to track your progress and remind yourself how far you've come. Looking back at these visual recollections can be quite motivational and encouraging.

• **Set new goals:** Use your achievements as a springboard to set new, more demanding goals for yourself. Having something to aspire for will help you stay motivated and engaged throughout your trip.

• **Be kind to yourself:** Throughout your journey, celebrate not only your accomplishments but also your efforts and endurance. Recognize that failures are a normal part of the process and that any progress, no matter how tiny, is worth celebrating.

Remember that celebrating your accomplishments is a crucial part of keeping momentum and staying inspired on your journey. Take the time to celebrate your accomplishments and slap yourself on the back for all of your hard work and devotion. You deserved it!

Continue Your Health and Wellness Journey

Your health and wellness journey is an ongoing one that takes commitment, effort, and endurance. Here are some pointers to help you stay on the path to a healthier lifestyle:

• **Stay focused on your goals:** Remember why you began your trip in the first place. Visualize your success and use it as inspiration to continue pushing forward.

• **Embrace flexibility:** Life is full of unexpected difficulties and changes, so your approach to health and wellbeing must be fluid and adaptable. Don't be too hard on yourself if things don't go as planned; instead, change your path and keep pushing.

• **Prioritize self-care:** Incorporate self-care activities into your daily routine to nurture your body, mind, and spirit. This could involve exercising, meditation, spending time with loved ones, or engaging in hobbies that you enjoy.

• **Keep learning:** Maintain your curiosity and openness to new facts about health and fitness. Continuously educate yourself about diet, exercise, and mindfulness techniques to improve your comprehension and make more educated decisions.

• **Create a support network:** Surround yourself with friends, family members, or online communities that understand and support your health and fitness goals. A robust support network can help you stay accountable, motivated, and encouraged throughout your journey.

• **Practice gratitude:** Develop a grateful attitude toward your accomplishments and the chances that await you. Take time each day to concentrate on the good aspects of your health and fitness journey and show thanks for them.

• **Celebrate tiny victories:** Recognize and celebrate your accomplishments, no matter how minor. Every step forward is an opportunity to celebrate and be proud of oneself.

Remember that your health and wellness journey is unique to you; there is no one-size-fits-all solution. Trust yourself, listen to your body, and respect your unique needs and preferences as you continue on your path to health and happiness. You can attain your goals and live your best life by committing to them, being consistent, and loving yourself. Keep going; you got this!

Conclusion

Congratulations on finishing your journey through "Nutritious Cuisine for Weight Loss"! This book provided you with great insights into nutrition, weight loss programs, and practical recommendations for making healthier choices in a variety of scenarios. Armed with this knowledge, you're ready to embark on a long-term journey to better health and well-being. Remember that obtaining and maintaining a healthy weight is not about restriction or severe rules, but about striking a balance, eating a variety of nutritious meals, and listening to your body's signals. Whether you're cooking at home, dining out, or navigating social gatherings, you may make decisions that help you achieve your goals while also enjoying the delights of food and dining. As you progress, prioritize self-care, mindful nutrition, and regular physical activity to maintain your overall health and energy. Celebrate your accomplishments, learn from your setbacks, and remain dedicated to your road to a healthier, happier you.

Thank you for joining us on this voyage. Here's to a future full of tasty, nutritious meals and living life to the fullest!

www.ingramcontent.com/pod-product-compliance
Lightning Source LLC
Chambersburg PA
CBHW070754260726
48660CB00007B/3112